Everything You Need to Know About Acne

Causes ♦ Symptoms ♦ Treatment

Watch a video version:
https://www.youtube.com/watch?v=SXOWVDGprnY

By The Bizmove Health Team

Disclaimer

All the content found in this book was created for informational purposes only. The Content is not intended to be a substitute for professional medical advice, diagnosis, or treatment. Always seek the advice of your physician or other qualified health provider with any questions you may have regarding a medical condition. Never disregard professional medical advice or delay in seeking it because of something you have read in this book.

ISBN: 9798745300318

Everything You Need to Know About Acne

Acne is a common skin condition that happens when hair follicles under the skin become clogged. Sebum—oil that helps keep skin from drying out—and dead skin cells plug the pores, which leads to outbreaks of lesions, commonly called pimples or zits. Most often, the outbreaks occur on the face but can also appear on the back, chest, and shoulders.

Acne is an inflammatory disorder of the skin, which has sebaceous (oil) glands that connects to the hair follicle, which contains a fine hair. In healthy skin, the sebaceous glands make sebum that empties onto the skin surface through the pore, which is an opening in the follicle. Keratinocytes, a type of skin cell, line the follicle. Normally as the body sheds skin cells, the keratinocytes rise to the surface of the skin.

When someone has acne, the hair, sebum, and keratinocytes stick together inside the pore. This prevents the keratinocytes from shedding and keeps the sebum from reaching the surface of the skin. The mixture of oil and cells allows bacteria that normally live on the skin to grow in the plugged follicles and cause inflammation-swelling, redness, heat, and pain. When the wall of the plugged follicle breaks down, it spills the bacteria, skin cells, and sebum into nearby skin, creating lesions or pimples.

For most people, acne tends to go away by the time they reach their thirties, but some people in their forties and fifties continue to have this skin problem.

Who Gets Acne

People of all races and ages get acne, but it is most common in teens and young adults. When acne appears during the teenage years, it is more common in males. Acne can continue into adulthood, and when it does, it is more common in women.

Types of Acne

Acne causes several types of lesions, or pimples. Doctors refer to enlarged or plugged hair follicles as comedones. Types of acne include:

- Whiteheads: Plugged hair follicles that stay beneath the skin and produce a white bump.
- Blackheads: Plugged follicles that reach the surface of the skin and open up. They look black

on the skin surface because the air discolors the sebum, not because they are dirty.

- Papules: Inflamed lesions that usually appear as small, pink bumps on the skin and can be tender to the touch.
- Pustules or pimples: Papules topped by white or yellow pus-filled lesions that may be red at the base.
- Nodules: Large, painful solid lesions that are lodged deep within the skin.
- Severe nodular acne (sometimes called cystic acne): Deep, painful, pus-filled lesions.

Causes of Acne

Doctors and researchers believe that one or more of the following can lead to the development of acne:

- Excess or high production of oil in the pore.
- Buildup of dead skin cells in the pore.
- Growth of bacteria in the pore.

The following factors may increase your risk for developing acne:

- **Hormones.** An increase in androgens, which are male sex hormones, may lead to acne. These increase in both boys and girls normally during puberty and cause the sebaceous glands to enlarge and make more sebum. Hormonal changes related to pregnancy can also cause acne.

- **Family history.** Researchers believe that you may be more likely to get acne if your parents had acne.
- **Medications.** Certain medications, such as medications that contain hormones, corticosteroids, and lithium, can cause acne.
- **Age.** People of all ages can get acne, but it is more common in teens.

The following do not cause acne, but may make it worse.

- Diet. Some studies show that eating certain foods may make acne worse. Researchers are continuing to study the role of diet as a cause of acne.
- Stress.
- Pressure from sports helmets, tight clothes, or backpacks.
- Environmental irritants, such as pollution and high humidity.
- Squeezing or picking at blemishes.
- Scrubbing your skin too hard.

Diagnosis of Acne

To diagnose acne, health care providers may:

- Ask about your family history, and, for girls or women, ask about their menstrual cycles.
- Ask you about your symptoms, including how long you have had acne.
- Ask what medications you are currently taking or recently stopped.
- Examine your skin to help determine the type of acne lesion.
- Order lab work to determine if another condition or medical disorder is causing the acne.

Treatment for Acne.

The goal of treatment is to help heal existing lesions, stop new lesions from forming, and prevent scarring. Medications can help stop some of the causes of acne from developing, such as abnormal clumping of cells in the follicles, high sebum levels, bacteria, and inflammation. Your doctor may recommend over-the-counter or prescription medications to take by mouth or apply to the skin.

Topical medications, which you apply to the skin, include:

- Antibiotics, which are usually used with other topical medications. Benzoyl peroxide, which kills bacteria and may decrease the production of sebum.

- Resorcinol, which can help break down blackheads and whiteheads.
- Retinoids, which come from vitamin A and can help treat lesions and reduce inflammation. They can also help prevent the formation of acne and help with scarring.
- Salicylic acid, which helps break down blackheads and whiteheads and also helps reduce the shedding of cells lining the hair follicles.
- Sulfur, which helps break down blackheads and whiteheads.

Topical medicines come in many forms, including gels, lotions, creams, soaps, and pads. In some people, topical medicines may cause side effects such as skin irritation, burning, or redness. Talk to your doctor about any side effects that you experience.

For some people, the doctor may prescribe oral medications, such as:

- Antibiotics, which help slow or stop the growth of bacteria and reduce inflammation. Doctors usually prescribe antibiotics with other topical therapies and usually for moderate to severe acne, such as severe nodular acne (also called cystic acne).
- Retinoids, which work through the blood stream to help treat acne and open up the pore. This

allows other medications, such as antibiotics, to enter the follicles and treat the acne. Similar to topical retinoids, taking the medication by mouth can also help prevent the formation of acne and help with scarring

- Hormone therapy, used primarily in women, which helps stop the effects of androgens on the sebaceous gland.
- Corticosteroids, which help lower inflammation in severe acne, including severe nodular acne. Your doctor may recommend injecting the medication directly into affected areas of your skin.

Some people who have severe acne that does not respond to topical or oral medications may need additional treatments, such as:

- Laser and light therapies. However, researchers are still studying the best types of light and the amount needed to treat acne.
- Procedure to remove the acne when other treatments are not helpful.
- Superficial chemical peels that a doctor recommends and applies to the area.
- Surgical procedures to help treat and repair scarring.

Who Treats Acne

The following health care providers may diagnose and treat acne:

- Dermatologists, who specialize in conditions of the skin, hair, and nails.
- Primary health care providers, including family doctors, internists, or pediatricians.

Living With Acne

If you have acne, the following recommendations may help you in taking care of your skin.

- Clean your skin gently. Use a mild cleanser in the morning, in the evening, and after heavy exercise. Try to avoid using strong soaps, astringents, or rough scrub pads. Rinse your skin with lukewarm water.
- Shampoo your hair regularly. If you have oily hair, you may want to wash it every day.
- Avoid rubbing and touching skin lesions. Squeezing or picking blemishes can cause scars or dark blotches to develop.
- Shave carefully. Make sure the blade is sharp, and soften the hair with soap and water before applying shaving cream. Shave gently and only when necessary to reduce the risk of nicking blemishes.

- Use sunscreen, and avoid sunburn and suntan. Many of the medicines used to treat acne can make you more prone to sunburn.
- Choose cosmetics carefully. All cosmetics and hair care products should be oil free. Choose products labeled noncomedogenic, which means they do not clog pores. In some people, however, even these products may make acne worse.

Acne can cause embarrassment or make you feel shy or anxious. If you have any of these feelings, talk to your doctor.

326 Great Tips For Acne Cure

Acne can be painful, annoying, itchy, and drive you crazy. However if you don't like the amount of acne you have you can take steps to reduce or even eliminate your acne. By following the information that you will find in this book you can achieve your dreams.

1. Try using lemons to combat acne breakouts. Some people find that lemon juice is very effective in getting rid of acne. If you have enlarged pores and oily skin, try applying lemon juice to the area. You should limit the use of lemon juice to only once or twice a week to avoid drying out your skin.

2. To get rid of unwanted acne, you may want to try a moisturizer. A lot of the face washes out there can actually dry out your skin. Always hydrate your face with water before applying the moisturizer. You can use a cream or lotion moisturizer to keep your skin looking and feeling great.

3. Wear a clean shirt to bed each night in order to avoid acne breakouts on your back, neck, and shoulders. Your nightshirt will absorb oils from your skin while you are sleeping. If you wear the same shirt again the next night, you will be putting these oils back on your skin. Wearing clean shirts each night avoids this problem.

4. When you are in the shower and washing your hair, tilt your head back when cleaning off your shampoo. Shampoo can sometimes stick to your face after your shower, irritating your skin and creating more acne. Alternatively, you can wash your hair in the sink to establish more control and eliminate the soap from hitting your face.

5. Everybody gets pimples, but the worst thing to do is pop them. Popping zits can leave scarring, redness, or cause swelling. When you pop a pimple, you are just pushing the infection back into the skin, and really making it a lot worse. Be kind to your skin and no matter how embarrassing it may be, don't pop your pimples.

6. Change your pillowcase everyday. Oil, bacteria, sweat and other impurities can build up on your pillowcase. Then, every time you lie down on your bed these impurities are transferred onto your skin and can cause acne outbreaks. If you

don't have many pillowcases use a clean towel over your pillow instead.

7. If over-the-counter treatments haven't improved your acne breakouts, a dermatologist can prescribe more advanced treatments. A cream that might be prescribed for you is Retin-A, which you apply to your skin daily. While effective for many patients, it's important to understand that it does take several weeks to achieve improvement.

8. In addition to other dietary changes you can make to target acne, consider reducing your red meat intake. Red meat is often cultivated with growth hormones. These hormones, when ingested, can disrupt your body's natural physiologic balance. This causes problems with your immune system and strips your skin of its natural defenses.

9. Easier said than done, but a good way to keep skin cleaner and less acne prone is to keep your hands off of it. As you use your hands throughout the day they gather all kinds of grime, oil and other unmentionables. Touching your face adds unnecessary contaminants that your skin must then contend with so wash your

hands often and avoid face contact whenever possible.

10. An important tip to consider when concerning acne is to avoid drastic temperature changes with foods and beverages. This is important because too hot or cold temperatures can actually cause acne to occur around the mouth. This is not something that common, however it is something to watch out for if nothing else works.

11. If you have marks from acne scars or burns, one of the best things that you can do is massage the area that is red. Massaging your skin helps to improve circulation, which will expedite the healing process of your scars. Massage your scar several times a day for optimal results.

12. Avoid touching or popping pimples. When you pop pimples you spread the bacterium from inside the pimple to more pores. You increase the likelihood of more pimples as a result. Touching the pimples can be just as bad, as you bring dirt and germs to the face through contact with your hands. Treat them with medicine and adopt a hands off plan.

13. Always use moisturizer. Most topical acne medications that are available contain ingredients that dry out the skin. A good moisturizer will minimize skin peeling and dryness, preventing further damage from occurring. If possible, select a gel-based moisturizer, as this will not add any extra oil to your skin which can clog pores.

14. Drink a lot of water. Water can help to reduce the amount of acne. Water helps by flushing the toxins out of your body. The more water you drink, the more the built-up toxins get diluted from your body and flushed out. A good amount of water to aim for is around 6-8 cups a day.

15. To combat acne make sure you wash your face with warm water at least twice a day- in the morning when getting ready to start your day and at night before going to bed. Washing with warm water helps clear pores of dirt and dead skin that can accumulate overnight and during the day.

16. Make sure that you do not over wash your face. You should wash your face using a mild soap and then gently pat it try. If you scrub it too much or use a strong soap it could further irritate your acne and make your face look even worse then it was.

17. Make a fresh mint paste. This is known as an effective way to fight acne problems. You can grind up fresh mint into a powder and mix with water. You can either use this as a mask for the whole face or apply it to areas affected with acne to help clear it up.

18. Did you know that acne can be caused by allergies? Allergies are a natural reaction that your immune system uses to fight off something that is trying to work it's way to inside your body. The problem is, your body can sometimes end up fighting things it just doesn't need to, because it was incorrectly programmed to do so. An allergy specialist can help by testing to find what allergies you do have. It could be something simple, such as dairy, or it could be more complex such as the paraffin wax in your hairspray. If your allergies are bad enough, an allergist can even give you shots that help to reprogram you body so that it no longer fights the things it doesn't need to fight.

19. Washing your face daily is a very important in preventing acne. It removes oil from your skin and also dead skin from the face. Be sure not to scrub your face too harshly, a gentle washing is all that you need. Make sure that the clothes and towels that you use are clean!

20. When it comes to acne the biggest tip that anyone can offer is try not to touch your face. In studies it's been show that the average person touches their face thousands of times a day. Just imagine all the bacteria, dirt, and grime on your hands. So if you want to be acne free, the first step to take is to keep your hands away from your face.

21. For girls whose acne is brought on by hormonal issues, then starting a birth control regimen can be very effective in fighting those blemishes. Only a doctor can prescribe them to you, so make sure you seek the advise of a medical doctor. By putting your body on a regular hormone cycle, it can clear up those breakouts.

22. Don't give up on medications too soon. Acne treatments can take anywhere from 2 to 6 weeks to improve your skin and some can cause your skin to look worse before it looks better. Be patient and give a new treatment at least a month before giving up on it.

23. Treat stubborn acne with care. Abrasive cleansers may seem like they're getting the job done, but you may be irritating your skin, which leads to further breakouts. By exfoliating too

often, you are triggering your skin to create an excess of oil. This builds up quickly in irritated, puffy pores, making the perfect recipe for new blemishes.

24. In order to prevent breakouts, try to incorporate more Zinc into your diet. It is necessary for the skin's oil producing glands and an essential antibacterial mineral. It is proven that a person whose diet is low in Zinc is more likely to develop both acne and blackhead outbreaks on their face.

25. If you are concerned that your acne does not seem to be going away, make a paste by mixing cinnamon powder and honey. Put the paste on your face before you fall asleep and use warm water to rinse it away in the morning. It will not only help your acne, but it will nourish your skin, as well.

26. If you are using an acne treatment on your blemishes, make sure to put the product on both your face and your neck. This technique ensures that you are treating any area that could potentially be problematic for your skin. It will also keep your current situation from worsening.

27. An important tip to consider when concerning acne is that if you have a blemish that you do not have time to wait for it to heal on its own, consider some creative makeup techniques to cover it up. This is important so that you allow proper time for healing, and allow yourself to go about your life.

28. Changing your diet is a great way to control acne. Eating fresh fruits and vegetables and including nuts and seeds in your everyday meals will help fix any deficiencies you might have in vitamins and minerals that help keep acne away. Fruits also have been known to help overall skin appearance, giving you a radiant glow.

29. An important tip to consider for treating acne is to use tea tree oil. This can prove to be a great, natural way to clear up acne or pimples. Tea tree oil will kill the bacteria that responsible for causing pimples and will help to rid you of acne. Be sure to only apply to the concerned area and apply with either a cotton ball or swab.

30. The age old wisdom that touching your face makes acne worse is actually true, so stop it! Your hands pick up all kinds of nasty germs during the day, and the more you pick at your face, the more you open up your skin to let those

bugs inside. Bacteria causes zits, so don't let any get on your face!

31. Increase your vitamin A and beta carotene intake to help stop acne. Both of these nutrients, taken as supplements or eaten in foods which are high in their content, help to make skin healthier and strengthen your immune system. Try eating some cantaloupe and carrots, or kale and spinach, to get the levels you need to clear up your skin.

32. For men shaving not only has a huge impact on their appearance, but also on the health of their skin. Razors, even while being run through water, can become dirty, and when rubbing against skin (expecting the pores to be opened with warm water ahead of time), will easily create an opportunity for acne to arise.

33. Acne can be treated efficiently by a professional dermatologist. If your insurance covers dermatology visits, or you have the finances to pay on your own, you should go see a dermatologist. Dermatologists have deep knowledge about all types of skin problems and will select the most effective, medical-grade techniques to treat your specific type of acne.

34. Maintaining an active lifestyle is beneficial in so many ways. Activity causes sweat however, and sweat that lingers on the skin can cause acne flare ups. Always use a mild cleanser after exercising to keep the skin clean and free of dried sweat. A gentle exfoliant once or twice a week can also help.

35. Sometimes acne can be severe and you need to seek treatment from a licensed Dermatologist. Your Dermatologist can prescribe medications, skin care products, and surgery which would not be available over the counter. Seeking treatment sooner, rather than later, can allow for the most effective cure.

36. Tretinoin, a topical retinoid, is a popular medication used to treat comedonal acne, blackheads and whiteheads. It is the acid form of vitamin A and works by increasing skin cell turnover and clearing blocked pores. The medication is available in cream or gel from under the following brand names: Stieva-A, Aberela, Atralin, Airol, Retin-A, Avita, Refissa and Renova.

37. Eat one to two tablespoons of pumpkin seeds a day in order to prevent acne breakouts. Pumpkin seeds are a good source of zinc, an essential

mineral. Recent studies show that many people who suffer from acne breakouts are zinc deficient. Snack on pumpkin seeds throughout the day for spotless skin.

38. A great way to prevent acne is to keep your bedding clean. This is especially important for your pillowcase which can absorb the sweat, oil and tears that you naturally produce during the night. Your face sleeps on this every day so it is imperative that it be clean. Keeping it clean will prevent a lot of breakouts in the future.

39. If you are using all of the over the counter products on the market to no avail, try washing your face with only water. This will guarantee that no soap residue sticks to your skin, as you will have a better chance of maintaining a healthy palette and reducing blemishes.

40. To keep acne to a minimum, it is best to keep your hands clean and to avoid touching or scratching your face. Dirty hands can create black heads filled with dirt and white heads filled with pus. Dirt, not only comes from your hands, but from linen, as well. Make sure to wash your bed sheets and pillow cases regularly. If you consciously think about how many hours your

face is in contact with the pillow, you won't forget to clean the pillowcases!

41. Clean your cell phone and house phones regularly to avoid acne breakouts. Gently clean the screen and number pad with a damp cotton swap and some rubbing alcohol. This will remove any left over bacteria and oils from the surface and won't reapply them to your cheek and ear, when you go to talk.

42. It is true that workouts are good for you, but they may also lead to new acne. This is why it is important to shower after your workout. Showering removes the sweat, dirt, oil and bacteria left behind after the workout, which could encourage new acne to form if not removed.

43. Acne is a natural bodily response. You should never invest in a product that you see on the internet or that you see on TV that guarantees your acne will go away in an hour. These products almost always are all hype, which will leave you without money and with acne.

44. To help improve your acne problem avoid excessive sun exposure. A small amount of sun exposure is healthy for the skin and a light tan

will help to hide some of the redness associated with acne. Too much exposure to sunlight, however, will cause skin to shed more than normal, resulting in clogged pores and an eventual increase in acne.

45. To decrease your acne breakouts, consider what types of things you are putting in your hair. Gels, sprays and oils can move onto your face very easily which then lead to clogged pores and skin irritations. It's best, if you are prone to acne, to stick with a mild shampoo and conditioner.

46. To battle acne, wash the things that often come into contact with your body. Frequently wash things like washrags, towels, sheets and pillowcases. Pillowcases, sheets and washcloths often collect bacteria which can cause acne. If you do not regularly wash your clothing it can also cause acne.

47. If you have problems with acne, it may be a symptom of a lack of nutrients. Try to eat healthy food, and take a daily multivitamin. If your skin lacks the nutrition it needs, it often fights back by producing excess oils and clogging pores, leading to acne symptoms.

48. Consider taking a probiotic. If you have been prescribed an antibiotic by your doctor or dermatologist either directly for your acne or due to an illness it is important to replace the good bacteria in your body. Antibiotics destroy all the bacteria in your digestive system both the good and the bad. This can lead to constipation as well as absorbing less of important vitamins and nutrients. Between the vitamin deficiencies and built up toxins, antibiotics can sometimes cause an even worse acne breakout. Probiotics replace the helpful good bacteria that you have lost.

49. To help keep acne away try to keep your hands away from your face. Our hands stay dirty. When you touch your face you are putting bacteria and dirt on your face which has the potential to clog your skin's pores. The dirt and bacteria that clogs the pores can lead to pimples.

50. You can avoid acne issues by changing your bed linens regularly. When you sleep at night, the dead skin cells can actually get caked into your pores. The longer the sheets go without being washed, the more bacteria is going to be on them and the more likely you are to have a breakout.

51. To avoid getting acne, you should drink a lot of water. Drinking enough water allows you to

sweat: sweating helps clean up your pores and get rid of the oil that causes your skin to break out. Make sure you drink at least eight glasses of water a day, especially in the summertime.

52. If you want to avoid breakouts, eat more beta-carotene, also known as vitamin A. This vitamin is a core ingredient in the structure of your skin, meaning your body needs it to produce skin cells, as well as for cell growth. Vitamin A also helps promote immune response, which helps heal existing acne faster. You can get more vitamin A by eating foods like carrots, spinach, bell peppers, basil and tomatoes.

53. To help rid your skin of acne, drink at least 8 glasses of water a day. Drinking water can help carry the waste material that causes acne and blackheads out of your body and work to flush out your skin. This will help clear your skin of blemishes and blackheads.

54. If you feel that your acne is very severe, you can see a dermatologist for potential antibiotics to help your skin from the inside out. Minocycline is one of the best oral treatments that you can take, as it will kill the bacteria that is causing your pimples and redness.

55. One thing you want to do to avoid acne breakouts is to avoid tanning booths. These cause an unnatural buildup of pigment in your skin and release chemicals on the surface of your skin. This causes more blockage of oils in your pores, which leads to further acne breakouts.

56. Prevent breakouts with this easy tip. Clean your cellphone (and desktop phone at work) thoroughly with an alcohol wipe each day to take off excess oils. When you press your face against these objects, your pores can become clogged with old residue. When you don't clean these devices, you put yourself at risk to breakouts.

57. In the winter, try to avoid places that typically contain dry air. When there is little moisture in the air you are around, there is a good chance for your skin to react negatively and dry out. This can lead to excess acne and red blemishes, due to the irritation that dryness causes.

58. As hard as it may be, do not touch your face with your hands unless you have washed them first. The bacteria and oils on your hands, rub onto your face and are often contributing factors toward common skin problems. You can carry around hand sanitizer and use that if you are on

the go, rather than stopping somewhere to wash your hands.

59. Buy non-comedogenic moisturizers, but be careful about the claims these moisturizers often make. These moisturizers typically help prevent acne but companies are not required by law to prove that the moisturizers actually work. Sometimes companies exaggerate their claims. Try the product on your skin to see if it is a good fit for you.

60. It is important not to vigorously scrub the affected area when you have acne. This will just irritate your skin and make your acne even worse. Also, try to limit washing the affected area to only two washings each day. Remember, acne is not caused by practicing poor hygiene.

61. Avoid caffeine to keep your skin nice and clear. Caffeine triggers your body to produce more stress hormones. Stress hormones will cause your body to react in ways that will increase the amount of acne flare-ups. Stay away from caffeine containing products to help clear up your acne issues.

62. For athletes who struggle with acne, remember that sweat can clog your pores and increase

break-outs. To mitigate damage to your skin caused by lingering sweat (especially from helmet buckles and pressing football chin-straps), wipe your face as often as possible while playing. Also, try to gain access to water and rinse your face, as time allows.

63. Antibiotics are good for fighting acne, but it is best to take pro-biotic or pre-biotic supplements along with them. Antibiotics have a negative impact on the healthy bacteria that assist with digestion. Pre-biotics and probiotics counteract this side effect. Healthy digestion is a significant factor in preventing acne outbreaks, so these supplements will help antibiotics work better.

64. Ask your dermatologist if he or she feels that prescribing topical retinoids like Tazorac, Avita, or tretinoin are a good option to treat your severe acne. These substances effectively penetrate the skin to normalize skin cell functions, which then allows your pores to remain clear of acne-irritating dead skin cells.

65. One of the easiest, most effective, and affordable ways to noticeably improve the appearance, texture, and tone of your skin is to stay consistently hydrated by consuming water instead of sugary colas or fruit juices. Keeping

your body hydrated can help your skin stay acne-free by maintaining balance and moisture from within.

66. If you have acne and long hair or bangs you need to keep your hair away from and off of your face. The oil in your hair will get on your face and cause or contribute to any breakouts. It's also best to wash your hair at least everyday and also after working out.

67. Try to treat your acne early. Many serious cases of acne got that way because treatment did not start until much later. At the first sign of a breakout, you should take steps to stop it before it gets worse. This means gentle cleansing, keeping hydrated, eating well, exercising and sleeping well. When in doubt, see a physician or dermatologist.

68. If you are suffering from acne, try to be aware of things that may transfer bacteria to your problem areas. For example, be sure to clean your cell phone regularly if you tend to hold it against your face. This will help prevent those unnecessary breakouts, and lead you one step closer to problem-free skin!

69. A good way to relieve those acne problems is to use something that originally comes from down under. Tea tree oil is a great remedy that can clear up problem zits in no time. Buy it at your favorite drugstore and just dab some on a cotton ball and apply to the problem areas.

70. A great way to treat breakouts is to save your used chamomile tea bags and apply them to problem areas on your face. They will help soothe and control acne. This is a great way to treat acne as it's cheap, natural and effective, and you are using something you likely already have at home.

71. Don't suffer alone. See a dermatologist. While many people have minor breakouts or pimples, those with true and severe acne should seek the advise of a professional. They will be able to give you the best possible defense against it with treatments, cleansers, and when necessary, prescription medications.

72. If you are an otherwise healthy adult woman with serious acne issues, consider asking your doctor if birth control pills could facilitate the problem. Birth control pills help regulate your hormone levels and most acne breakouts in young adults are related to hormone fluctuations.

The regulation of hormones could reduce the number of breakouts you suffer.

73. There are a variety of foods that can help your body prevent the formation of acne. Some of these foods include seafood, poultry and whole grains. These foods also keep your body running well. If you want to give your body the upper hand against acne, then make sure you eat these prescribed foods.

74. If you have deep, cystic acne, you may find that over-the-counter medications aren't very helpful. A dermatologist may prescribe Accutane for these kinds of cases. Accutane is a powerful medication that is taken as a pill, and generally is not prescribed lightly. If your doctor feels this is the right treatment for you, be sure to take it exactly as prescribed, and always report any side effects to your physician.

75. If you're struggling with acne, reconsider your diet. If you eat a lot of fried and greasy food, your skin may end up producing extra oil in response. Add more fresh fruits and vegetables in your daily diet. Try eliminating processed sugars found in candy bars. If you have any food allergies, steer clear of foods that cause them!

76. You can create a facial mask by crushing aspirin and putting it thinly on your face. Aspirin contains salicylic acid which is great for treating acne. As you are not using the aspirin for its intended purpose, it is advised that you speak with a doctor before starting this method.

77. If you are having trouble with acne, pick up some garlic pieces the next time you are at the grocery store. Try rubbing them directly on your blemishes. You can also treat the skin around the pimple as well. After several applications, you should notice a difference in your skin.

78. Baking soda can be used for gentle, acne-friendly exfoliation. A paste of baking soda and water will give a boost to the body's natural exfoliating action. It is especially good for acne-infected areas because it is less harsh than most abrasive exfoliating products. Be careful not to confuse baking powder with baking soda, though!

79. To help treat excessively oily areas of the skin, which can be prone to acne, try a potato facial. Cut a raw potato into thin slices and place the slices in oil-rich areas of the face, such as the forehead and chin. Gently rub the slices against the skin so that the potato juice saturates the

skin. Leave the potato slices on face for at least twenty minutes, then gently rinse the face with water.

80. Heat and light therapy can sometimes be used effectively to treat acne. This treatment involves applying intense heat to the skin, while also using a strong light source. The process clears the skin of bacteria and cuts down the size of some glands as well. The method should only be performed by a licensed Dermatologist.

81. If you are struggling with acne, it is important that you wash your face in the morning and sometime at night close to when you will go to bed. The importance of this is that this keeps the pores from getting clogged with the dirt and oils on your face, thus keeping your face acne free!

82. Banish your acne the natural way by treating your face with Tea Tree Oil after washing your face. This non-abrasive treatment naturally occurs in Australian trees, and is a natural alternative to harsher over-the-counter products. It is available at health food stores nationwide. As a natural antiseptic, Tea Tree Oil can be just as effective as salicylic acid in treating acne. It can also treat wounds.

83. To clear up and prevent acne, increase your zinc intake. There's been recent evidence, showing that too little zinc in your diet, can actually be a cause of acne. Zinc also helps prevent acne with its antibacterial properties, is essential to the immune function that heals pimples and helps your body's cells (including skin cells) to function properly. Foods rich in zinc include, shiitake and crimini mushrooms, asparagus, collard greens, maple syrup and shrimp.

84. During the course of the day, try to maximize your fruit and vegetable intake to control acne. Vegetables are great for your skin and can supply your body with the nutrients necessary to eliminate free radicals internally. Complement your breakfast, lunch or dinner with an infusion of fruits or vegetables for clear skin.

85. Often foods will be the culprit of the acne that you have on your skin. If you notice that a specific food is causing your acne, try to limit it as much as possible. Ice cream, milk, cheese and other dairy products have been shown to increase acne.

86. If you ever pop a pimple, make sure that you put Neosporin on it as soon as possible. Neosporin helps aid the healing process and can

accelerate a scab so that you do not scar as easily. Once the scab is formed, never pick at it, as this can impede the healing process.

87. If you have a project that is due for school, do not wait until the last minute, which can cause stress and anxiety. Plan in advance and finish ahead of time, to avoid unnecessary stress the night before it is due. This will help you feel comfortable during the day and reduce breakouts at college.

88. Make sure to get a lot of sleep. Whenever you get sleep reduce the amount of stress on your skin. This reduces the amount of blockage in your pores and decreases the amount of blackheads you will get. It also decreases the amount of breakouts you will get.

89. If you have very severe acne and it is affecting your daily life, then a visit to a dermatologist is advised. A dermatologist can prescribe an oral antibiotic or an adapalene gel. These medications can treat severe acne, but their use needs to be monitored by a health care professional, as side effects can occur.

90. Drink lots of water to help get rid of acne. When your skin is dehydrated it can't effectively

get rid of the dead skin cells, which can then clog up your pores and cause acne. It is recommended that you drink at least two liters, or half a gallon, of still mineral water every single day to keep the acne away.

91. Be careful about wearing hats. The sun is bad for your skin. Hats can be great protection from the sun. Unfortunately, they can also cause you to sweat around your hairline. Sweat clogs pores and can cause you to break out. If you seem to be breaking out around your hairline often, it might be time to leave the hat at home for a while.

92. When you are done with exercising, make it a point to hit the shower. Sweating and sloughing dirt and dead skin out of your pores is great, however, not showering before the sweat has time to dry will cause your pores to be clogged with the same refuse that you cleared out. Rest for five or ten minutes then get in the shower and wash it away.

93. Stress is one of the most common contributors of acne breakouts. The reason for this is that stress causes the release of a hormone called cortisol. Cortisol is known to intensify acne. It can cause relatively small acne problems to turn

into severe breakouts. You should therefore try to stay conscious of your stress levels and regularly engage in stress relieving activities such as exercise or meditation.

94. If you have bad acne scars, you may want to consider visiting a plastic surgeon! They have certain methods, such as laser treatments, that cannot be bought or found in a pharmacy. Although this can be a pricey option, it is also the most effective one for getting rid of acne scars!

95. Eat lots of carrots, dried apricots, sweet potatoes, and spinach to help manage your acne. All of these fruits and vegetables contain large portions of Vitamin A. Vitamin A is an amazing antioxidant. It can help to rid your body of toxins and repair skin tissue as well.

96. A good tip concerning acne is to not fret too much about having oily skin. Some people are just destined to have oily skin, while others will enjoy having normal skin. You must learn to accept your skin for the way it is and realize there's no magic fix.

97. To minimize facial acne, be sure to wash your skin twice a day, not less and not more. Natural

beneficial oils may be washed away with more frequent washing. A morning and an evening wash with a mild cleanser should wash away enough excess oil to keep acne at bay.

98. If you have acne prone skin, change your pillowcase frequently. Over time, dirt and oil from your hair and skin can build up on your pillowcase. When you lay your face down on it at night it can then clog your pores, leading to acne. The best way to avoid this problem is by regularly changing your pillowcase.

99. Acne can be treated efficiently by a professional dermatologist. If your insurance covers dermatology visits, or you have the finances to pay on your own, you should go see a dermatologist. Dermatologists have deep knowledge about all types of skin problems and will select the most effective, medical-grade techniques to treat your specific type of acne.

100.   Avoid spreading acne by not popping or forcing your pimples to drain. If you pop your pimples, you are spreading the very infection that causes the breakouts. This infection then spreads to other parts of your face causing more breakouts in more areas. Popping zits also can cause unnecessary redness, swelling and

permanent scarring, so it's best to leave them be and let them go away on their own or with acne medication.

101.   If you're fighting acne, check your moisturizers for ingredients that can make acne worse or prolong breakouts. Many rich or heavy moisturizing creams have ingredients that can clog pores, like sodium lauryl sulfate, cetearyl alcohol, cocoa butter or wheat germ oil. Other moisturizers contain ingredients like salicylic acid or retinol that can irritate skin that's trying to heal. Make sure to choose moisturizers that are non-comedogenic (non-clogging), non-acnegenic, and gentle on acne-prone skin.

102.   Putting lemon juice onto a cotton ball or cotton swab and applying the juice directly onto an acne scar or pimple, can be a great natural acne remedy. The citric acid dries out pimples and lightens red marks and scars. For sensitive skin, try diluting the lemon juice with water or honey before applying.

103.   If you are using all of the over the counter products on the market to no avail, try washing your face with only water. This will guarantee that no soap residue sticks to your skin, as you

will have a better chance of maintaining a healthy palette and reducing blemishes.

104.   When you shave, use minimal force if you are going over your acne. Try to use an electrical razor, so you do not have to go over your acne with a sharp blade. Electrical razors can minimize cutting, but may take a week or two for your body to get used to.

105.   When you are shopping for acne products in a drug store or mall, make sure that you purchase makeup that is designed specifically for acne. There are many foundations and concealers that are designed to fight acne while on your face, as opposed to a lot of products which exacerbate the problem.

106.   Vinegar is an effective home remedy for treating acne. Simply apply white or distilled vinegar on the affected area and leave it there for 10 minutes. The vinegar will get rid of the bacteria which is causing the acne. Make sure to dilute the vinegar with a small amount of lukewarm water before applying it to the affected skin surface.

107.   To keep your skin clear and keep your diet on track at the same time, drink plenty of water

every day. While most people think of water intake as a dietary tip, keeping your body hydrated is also crucial to keeping your skin clean and clear. Simultaneously cutting back on sugary drinks like soda will also cut back on breakouts.

108.   Use a cucumber to help you to get rid of unsightly blemishes. Mix the cucumber up into a paste and apply it like a mask on your face. Allow it to sit for approximately one hour. Not only will it help with your pimples, but it is a nice, soothing remedy for your skin as well.

109.   Clearing up acne can be as easy as avoiding refined carbohydrates and sugar. Pasta, white bread, rice and sugar, are all known for causing a myriad of problems and recently, they have been indicated as a cause of acne. They can also cause a surge in insulin which can lead to Type II Diabetes and hormone imbalance, which can cause pimples to appear.

110.   You can use a natural mask of water and baking soda, mixed to a paste-like consistency, 3 times weekly, to combat skin breakouts. You should cleanse your face first, but don't use toner or rinse with cold water. Apply the baking soda and water paste to your face and leave it on for twenty minutes. Rinse it off with warm water

followed by a splash of cold water and a toner, if desired.

111.   If you are having difficulty with acne, wash your face two times a day. Make sure that you are not abrasive during the cleansing process; you do not want to harm your skin. Washing your face will help rid your skin of the sweat and oil that has been accumulating there. Just make sure not to overdo it; you do not want to dry out your skin.

112.   Stick to natural products if you have acne-prone skin. Many facial products contain harsh chemicals. These chemicals strip the skin of its natural oils. This causes your skin to become dry, or in some cases, actually triggers an increase in oil production in the face to compensate for the lost oils. Both outcomes often result in even more acne.

113.   Here is a way of treating acne that is a little bit off the wall. You want to mix cut up strawberries with sour cream and make sure it is blended well. Then apply the mixture to your face like a beauty mask. This mixture will cool your face and clear up problem areas.

114.   To eliminate acne, one of the best things that you can do is exercise at least three times per week. Exercising helps to eliminate toxins from the inside out, which can build up under your skin and cause irritation and acne lesions. Additionally, exercising facilitates sweat, unclogging your pores and creating a pristine look.

115.   Just like with bleaching your hair in the sun, putting lemon juice on your skin can lighten the redness associated with acne, and help to lighten the old scars left behind as well. Just dab some on your breakouts with a cotton swab. Be careful that you don't overdue it as some people say that it can sting and burn a bit.

116.   To limit the formation of acne, try to reduce the amount of ketchup and tomato sauce that you consume. These foods have a lot of sugar and carbohydrates and can kick start the formation of acne. Try to stick to natural foods that are raw and organic to eliminate acne through your diet.

117.   Add water to your moisturizer if it feels thick and heavy. People with oily skin need to avoid a heavy moisturizer that will make their skin even more oily. If you are suffering from acne even

after routinely using moisturizer, mix a drop of water into the dollop of moisturizer before you put it on your face.

118.   If you are trying to get rid of acne, you may think that you need to wash your face a lot. However, you need to make sure that you do not over do it. If you apply harsh chemicals to your face over and over, it can irritate your skin, only causing more acne.

119.   A great tip for covering up acne is by getting a tan. Acne and blemishes are much more noticeable on pale skin than on tan skin. Tanning outdoors for at least ten minutes each day can go a long way in covering up that acne that you're ashamed of.

120.   When you exercise, make sure to take a shower or bath, as soon as possible afterwards, to remove the sweat and oils that are produced. If you can, avoid wearing hats or helmets during a workout as that will cause you to sweat more, which can cause a flare up of your acne.

121.   Getting a little bit of sunshine every day helps prevent acne. Sunshine helps create Vitamin D in the body, which is an essential nutrient for the skin. However, do not stay in the

sun too long as this can create negative results for the skin. Taking a ten minute walk a day is sufficient.

122.   In order to prevent your acne from becoming more severe, you must never pop your pimples. When you pop your pimples, the bacteria clogged within your pores will be released, and can spread over the rest of your face resulting in greater inflammation and irritation. The bacteria on your hands can also intensify your acne.

123.   Be careful when shaving. If you are shaving and have an acne breakout, you can nick the acne, irritating the skin and potentially spreading bacteria to surrounding areas. To avoid this, moisten your beard thoroughly with soap and water prior to using shaving cream, use a sharp blade and shave slowly.

124.   For severe cases of acne, talk to your doctor about isotretinoin. Isotretinoin is a prescription oral medication, and it has been shown to be extremely effective in helping skin get clear and stay clear. There are serious side effects associated with the medication, particularly for pregnant women, so careful consideration is

needed to determine whether this is the right course of action for you.

125.   Do not allow sweat to linger after exercising. Gently wipe away sweat from the skin during exercise and use a mild face cleaner afterwards. Avoid cleansers that are alcohol based because they cause dry skin. By wiping sweat away during exercise and keeping your face clean your acne will improve.

126.   Get some sun. Too much sun is bad for your skin, however too little sun can be almost as bad. Sunlight triggers the creation of vitamin D in your body, and this vitamin is crucial for healthy skin. Not only will you have an increase in vitamin D, fresh air and sunshine can reduce stress another culprit in the fight against acne.

127.   Use skin care products and cosmetics that are oil free for preventing acne. The oils in these products can clog pores and increase outbreaks. These oils can also react negatively with your skin causing irritation and possible allergic reactions. Try to avoid oils in your hair care products, as well, because these can also come in contact with your skin and have the same effect.

128.   For controlling acne, don't use face washes or cleansers with oil or perfumes in them. Oil in these products can clog pores and cause new pimples to appear. Perfumes are not advised because they can burn or irritate the already sensitive, delicate skin associated with acne.

129.   If you have acne, be careful not to clean your skin too much! Daily cleansing is very important for healthy skin, but over-scrubbing irritates breakouts and does more harm than help. Cleansers can leave residues that may act as irritants as well. Lightly rubbing a gentle cleanser into your skin and rinsing well with water is the best way to fight off outbreaks.

130.   Avoid the sun during an acne breakout. The sun can damage your skin in many ways. You should especially avoid it during an acne breakout. Sunlight can make your acne much worse, increasing redness and causing inflammation. If you absolutely must be out in the sun for an extended period of time, remember to wear sunscreen.

131.   You can help keep acne away by washing your pillow case, at least every other day. Since your face lays on your pillow every night, oils and dirt from skin, get absorbed by your pillow

case. This oil and dirt then becomes redistributed on your skin, causing more breakouts.

132.   Lots of people get acne when they are stressed. Stress causes the body to produce the hormone cortisol, which may trigger acne outbreaks. By engaging yourself in activities that you find relaxing (such as deep breathing or yoga), you can greatly decrease your chances of having an acne outbreak.

133.   Avoiding acne can be as simple as just washing your pillow cases every other day. Every time you lay on your pillows, the case absorbs dirt and oils from your skin. The amount of time spent on your pillow helps reapply the dirt and oils that clog your pores leading to acne. Washing your pillow cases every other day, helps to keep your face clean.

134.   If you change your pillowcases and sheets often, you will avoid acne. Oils will collect on your pillow cases and sheets while you sleep. Then they can transfer them back to your skin. If you wash your linens frequently, you will be able to avoid this.

135.   You can treat acne scars on your face with a mild bleaching cream, many of which are

available over the counter at a local pharmacy. These creams take time to work, some as long as a couple of months, but if you stick with them the results are very much worth it. Once the scars are gone, you'll be able to see how much they detracted from the look of your skin.

136.   Touching your face can lead to more breakouts and blackheads. This is because your hands contain a lot of dirt and oils and you are just pouring that over the affected areas of your face. A mirror can be tempting to scratch and pick at your zits, but try and resist.

137.   Add water to your moisturizer if it feels thick and heavy. People with oily skin need to avoid a heavy moisturizer that will make their skin even more oily. If you are suffering from acne even after routinely using moisturizer, mix a drop of water into the dollop of moisturizer before you put it on your face.

138.   When trying to prevent acne, you should always use water-based, hypo allergenic makeup or moisturizer. These products are not guaranteed to prevent or help with acne. They are, however, less likely to increase your acne. Be sure to read all labeling on the products that you are buying to find out what is in it.

139.   One important step in the control of acne and other skin conditions is to eliminate as much stress from your life as possible. The hormones that your body produces when you are stressed can be detrimental to your health, body and skin. Reducing stress has so many benefits it is well worth the effort, be it by exercise, meditation or simply taking a few minutes a day to be alone with your favorite music. Stress has been shown to increase acne breakouts so make sure that your stress is under control.

140.   An important tip to consider concerning acne is to know why pimples and acne swell and contain puss. This is important to know because these are healthy reactions, showing that your body is fighting the infection. The swelling is caused by a mass of white blood cells, and the white puss is the result of those white blood cells doing their job then dying off.

141.   An important tip to consider when concerning acne is that once it starts to heal and enters the pimple stage, you need to keep a close eye on it. This is important because if treated incorrectly, this pimple may turn into a painful cyst that digs deep into your skin.

142.   An important tip to consider when concerning acne is that in addition to lotions, sun-tan lotions and sunscreens may also clog your pores. Be sure to choose the non-pore-clogging types, that will usually be labeled as such or state that they are non-comedgenic. It may help to check user reviews, as well.

143.   An important tip to consider concerning acne is to apply chamomile directly to your skin to try to cure it. This works great for acne and will make use of an item that you would have otherwise thrown away. After re-wetting a used tea bag, you may apply it directly to your acne and it will work to cure it.

144.   If you wear sunglasses, make sure that the lenses and the frames are cleaned every single week. Even though you can't see it, bacteria will build up on your sunglasses and contribute to acne formation. Clean your sunglasses often if you want to achieve bright, radiant skin around the eyes.

145.   Looking for a way to help you battle acne? Think about your caffeine intake and try to lower it. Caffeine can increase your stress levels which can then increase your oil production and then cause acne. Try to avoid things such as coffees,

sodas and chocolates and other products with caffeine stimulating ingredients.

146.   Consider taking a probiotic. If you have been prescribed an antibiotic by your doctor or dermatologist either directly for your acne or due to an illness it is important to replace the good bacteria in your body. Antibiotics destroy all the bacteria in your digestive system both the good and the bad. This can lead to constipation as well as absorbing less of important vitamins and nutrients. Between the vitamin deficiencies and built up toxins, antibiotics can sometimes cause an even worse acne breakout. Probiotics replace the helpful good bacteria that you have lost.

147.   Many women already know that cucumber slices can help get rid of bags under their eyes. But, not many know that it can help clear up acne as well. Grate a cucumber and apply it to any affected areas. Then sit back and relax for about fifteen minutes to let it do its work. Then, wash it away.

148.   Birth control can both be a cause and a preventative treatment for acne. For many adult women, going on the pill is to treat their adult acne. The pills contain hormones that can help the female's own hormones find balance and

some get clearer skin out of this. Many times though, when they get off of the pill, this can cause they're hormones to go haywire and they can start breaking out again.

149.   Try using witch hazel on your acne. Witch hazel is great at drawing out infection. It works well on acne as well. Just pour a little on a cotton ball and dab any area that is afflicted with acne. Feel free to repeat the process once a day or so.

150.   To get rid of acne, try not to have anything brush against your face repeatedly. Perhaps your hair cut causes your hair to touch your face and render it greasy. Avoid wearing scarves or hats, too. Do your best to keep your hands away from your face, especially if your hands are dirty.

151.   If you want to get rid of your acne, you should avoid wearing make up. Make up can conceal acne but it clogs your pores and may even irritate your skin. The chemicals contained in your makeup can also contribute to your skin breaking out. Remember that you do not need make up to be beautiful.

152.   To get rid of your acne, consider buying an anti-acne cream. You might have to try different brands to find one that works for you. Many

anti-acne creams are going to make your skin too dry or irritate it. You can compensate this by using a hydrating cream too.

153.   To help reduce your acne, be sure to use only natural skincare products. Many skincare products contain unnatural chemicals that can actually aggravate your skin, causing breakouts or making your acne worse. Stick to skincare products that have natural ingredients that will not irritate your skin, such as tea tree oil, a natural antibacterial.

154.   Use toothpaste to help your acne. This is a very effective home remedy for drying up pimples. Simply dab a small amount on the pimple, rub it in gently, and leave overnight. Upon waking, wash your face, and apply a little oil-free moisturizer to the area. You will definitely notice a difference. Two warnings when using toothpaste: only use the paste, not gel, and never apply toothpaste to broken skin.

155.   Limiting the amount of sugar and refined carbohydrates that you eat can help you reduce acne. These foods cause an increase in insulin and in something called IGF-1, both of which make your body produce an overabundance of male hormones. This encourages your skin to

produce a greasy substance that is a breeding ground for acne to form.

156.   For those who are looking for new ways or better ways to deal with their acne, the internet can be a very useful tool. For those who don't have access to the internet at home they can go to the public library. Online one can access a large database of helpful information.

157.   Chances are good that your acne is related to stress. It's important to take time each day to relax. Doing something that you like will reduce the stress and balance your hormones, which are the actual cause of acne. It is important to quit smoking and to limit the consumption of caffeine if you are prone to acne breakouts.

158.   Touching your face can lead to more breakouts and blackheads. This is because your hands contain a lot of dirt and oils and you are just pouring that over the affected areas of your face. A mirror can be tempting to scratch and pick at your zits, but try and resist.

159.   Resist the urge to pop or pick at pimples. Although it may feel like popping a pimple will get rid of it faster, it could make it much worse. Pinching will cause the skin to become more red

and swollen, and possibly, end up bleeding. This can cause scarring that will last forever, so be patient and let the pimple heal without popping.

160.   An important tip to consider when concerning acne is to consider taking a multi-vitamin supplement in addition to a healthy diet. This is important because acne can be a sign of many things, with malnutrition being one of them. If your body has all the nutrients it needs, then your skins natural oils will balance out.

161.   Exfoliate your skin once a week. It will remove the dead skin and buildup that will clog your pores and dull your complexion. Use scrubs that are specially formulated for the face and have tiny grains in it. Do not use the scrubs that have large seeds or grains in them because they will cause tears in your skin.

162.   Crush uncoated aspirin tablets and mix with water and then apply this mixture to the face to create an aspirin mask. Keep the aspirin mask on for about ten minutes. Aspirin contains salicylic acid that helps fade acne scars and helps to prevent future breakouts. When using an aspirin mask, aspirin can be absorbed into your bloodstream, so consult with your doctor before starting this skin care regiment.

163.　When trying to cure acne, stay away from alcohol, whether you consume it or use products containing alcohol. Alcohol's astringent properties work to strip away the top layer of the skin, this causes an increase in oil production. Oil works to clog your pores and cause blemishes and blackheads.

164.　You may also be intolerant of certain foods so be aware of this; if you notice you start to break out after you eat chocolate then don't eat chocolate for a while to see if this reduces your amount of acne. Each person is different, and you have to find what works for you.Remember that you are what you eat. In addition, try drinking more water and eating healthier foods as all of this will promote a healthy body.

165.　Shaving serves as exfoliation and therefore, can be an excellent way of removing dead skin cells. This can help to both prevent acne, and keep it from spreading if a break out has occurred. Avoid shaving any areas that are sore or infected however, as this can further irritate the skin.

166.　If back acne is an issue for you, then you may want to change your body cleanser. Opt for cleansers that contain salicylic acid or those geared toward clearing up acne and use these when you shower, once a day. Also, be sure to shower soon after vigorous exercise or physical activities, to avoid having the dirt and bacteria clog up your pores.

167.   To clear up acne, you should put a clean towel over your pillow every night. This stops bacteria from growing on your pillow, and it can really stop facial acne. Bacteria are a major cause of acne and avoiding them is an easy way to really clear up your face!

168.   If you breakout on your neck or body try a cleanser that has benzoyl peroxide. This ingredient helps to kill the excess bacteria that is on your skin and prevents future acne breakouts from forming. This product may yield excess redness so stop using if you see continuous irritation persisting.

169.   If you must continue to wear makeup during severe acne breakouts, try decontaminating your makeup sponges, brushes and applicators. This is a very simple procedure, just wash them and dip them in rubbing alcohol after each use and leave to air dry. This will help keep your applicators

clean, and rid them of oily residue left behind from oily skin.

170.   To help get rid of acne, eat more fresh fruits, vegetables, seeds and nuts. These foods contain essential vitamins and minerals that will boost your body's natural defenses against acne. Easy ways to get these into your diet are by making smoothies, drinking fruit juice or having a salad with your lunch or dinner.

171.   To avoid making your skin even more oily, avoid washing your face too many times a day in your pursuit to rid your skin of acne. Washing your face too often can lead to even oilier skin, which will of course worsen your acne instead of improving it. Wash your face once in the morning and once before bed.

172.   Getting a little bit of sunshine every day helps prevent acne. Sunshine helps create Vitamin D in the body, which is an essential nutrient for the skin. However, do not stay in the sun too long as this can create negative results for the skin. Taking a ten minute walk a day is sufficient.

173.   Stop touching your face. Your hands are host to all of the bacteria you pick up between

washings. Most of these bacteria are foreign to your physiology, making reactions a likely possibility. Furthermore, touching your face will make it harder to resist picking at blemishes. Blemishes need time and care, to heal without scarring.

174.   Many people with acne also have sensitive skin. The harsh ingredients in most medicines, topical treatments and washes can irritate the skin, causing more acne and redness than there was before. Find natural products and treatments that don't use chemicals. You can find many of these products in your local health food stores.

175.   Consider switching to a low-carb diet to improve your body's resistance to acne. While myths about chocolate causing acne are indeed untrue, do not assume that diet has no impact on your acne problems. Carbohydrates are relatively tough to digest. While your digestive system is working overtime on carbs, it can neglect other waste products. When these wastes build up in the skin, they contribute to the onset of acne.

176.   An important tip to consider when concerning acne is to try using a mixture of milk along with nutmeg directly on the area of concern. This is a great natural way to remove

acne from your skin. Apply enough of each ingredient in order to make a paste-like texture.

177.   An important tip to consider when concerning acne on your back is to wash your back up to twice a day. Depending on your oil production, this might be necessary to keep your back free from acne. If you do wash this frequently, be sure that you use a mild body wash or soap to prevent drying and irritation.

178.   While regularly applying sunscreen can protect your skin from aging prematurely, it can also lead to acne problems over time. The oils and compounds in popular sunblocks can clog enlarged pores, causing redness, irritation, and inflammation. Instead, opt for sunscreens that are labeled non-comedogenic, which means that they will not clog your pores.

179.   Keep your hands off your face. It might sound simple and a bit odd, but touching your face too often can actually make your skin break out. Your fingertips, especially, contain a lot of oil. Sitting with your hand on your face is a good habit to break if you are trying to improve your complexion.

180.   Be careful when shaving your face if you have acne. Try to use only a clean razor and avoid getting it and any cream or soap in or around any breakout. It can not only aggravate it, but a nick could leave it open to other kinds of infection that may cause further health problems.

181.   One of the most important ways to avoid getting acne is to keep your hands away from your face. The oils and bacteria on your fingers can actually damage your skin and cause pores to be clogged. Don't ever push on or irritate your face at all with your fingers.

182.   If you would like to reduce the size and color of your untimely breakouts, you may want to just try ice. The cooling effects will actually subside the swelling so the pimple is not as visible. Try icing before bed and you will wake up with a smaller, less noticeable pimple.

183.   To get rid of your acne, eat more fresh fruit and vegetables, as well as nuts and seeds. You can do this easily by having a smoothie with breakfast and eating a salad as a side dish with lunch or dinner. Brazil nuts are also great for controlling acne, as are pumpkin seeds.

184.   Friction and pressure can aggravate pimples and make them more likely to rupture which can cause scars. Avoid wearing tight clothing such as turtlenecks, holding a telephone to your cheek for too long and always adjust straps on helmets so they are not too restrictive. Try to wear clothing that breathes as well, such as cotton.

185.   Even though it is tempting to hide pimples on your face behind your hair, try not to let your hair touch your face. Oil, bacteria and styling products in your hair can be transferred onto your skin and aggravate your acne more. Headbands, Alice bands, clips and slides are great accessories that keep hair off your face.

186.   Do not touch your face. Because you use your hands to do almost everything, your hands carry much dirt, oil, and bacteria. To keep these contaminants from clogging your pores and causing breakouts, avoid touching your face unless absolutely necessary. If you must touch your face, wash your hands before.

187.   If you are suffering from acne, do not touch the areas affected by a breakout. Fingers transfer skin oils and dirt to acne-prone skin, exacerbating the problem and spreading infection. Unconscious face-touching gestures

should be eliminated. If you often rub your eyes or rest your chin on your hands, you are simply causing more problems for your skin.

188.   An important tip to consider when concerning acne is to know why your body has oil glands. This is important to know because while your oil glands can be your worst enemy when fighting acne, they are essential to your skin health. You oil glands are what lubricate your skin and keep it from drying out and cracking.

189.   Antibiotics are good for fighting acne, but it is best to take pro-biotic or pre-biotic supplements along with them. Antibiotics have a negative impact on the healthy bacteria that assist with digestion. Pre-biotics and probiotics counteract this side effect. Healthy digestion is a significant factor in preventing acne outbreaks, so these supplements will help antibiotics work better.

190.   Vitamin D is an essential component of not only reducing acne problems, but also having healthy skin in general. One amazing and free source of vitamin D is the sun! Make sure you spend some time outside on a daily basis. However, do not overdo it as the sun can be a

double edged sword. Staying out in the sun for an excessive amount of time and getting burnt is a cause of skin cancer.

191.   Honey and yogurt can make a great acne mask. Just mix one part honey to two parts yogurt. Apply to the entire face and leave on for about fifteen minutes. The yogurt has soothing properties and the honey has antiseptic properties. They are both wonderful for clearing your skin and keeping it fresh.

192.   One of the best ways to reduce acne is to reduce your stress levels. Stress causes oils and other things to stir up in your body which can then cause skin problems. Try things such as meditation or blogging or simply talking to a therapist to get yourself through stressful situations, and help you to de-stress so that your skin doesn't end up having to deal with the damaging effects.

193.   If you suffer from severe acne and no treatment has ever worked, you may want to see a dermatologist and ask for an accutane prescription. Accutane is the strongest acne drug available and can successfully clear your skin when nothing else has worked. Accutane has a

number of very serious side effects, so it should only be used as a last resort.

194.   It is important to remember not to touch acne prone skin with your hands on a frequent basis. Doing so will spread germs and infection, perhaps leading to worsening acne problems. Remember that acne prone skin is already sensitive and possibly broken. If you must touch it, do so with clean hands, and wash your hands afterwards.

195.   If you're just starting to break out, stop the acne spread before it gets worse. Even if you only have barely visible acne on your face, go to your local pharmacy and shop for some skin cleaning products. Those tailored to fight acne are best, but any product that cleans your pores works well, also.

196.   Get more vitamin A daily to have clearer skin free of breakouts. The beta-kerotene (a.k.a vitamin A) found in vegetables like carrots helps make the skin able to protect itself better against anything that could cause acne like dirt, oil, and foreign germs. It also helps make the skin repair itself more quickly.

197.   Make a mask of egg whites. Egg whites have been known to prevent acne in some instances. Try making a facial mask out of egg whites. Leave it on for fifteen to twenty minutes before washing it off. Alternatively, you can apply egg whites directly to pimples. This will often greatly reduce redness and swelling.

198.   Lots of people get acne when they are stressed. Stress causes the body to produce the hormone cortisol, which may trigger acne outbreaks. By engaging yourself in activities that you find relaxing (such as deep breathing or yoga), you can greatly decrease your chances of having an acne outbreak.

199.   Cucumbers are a great natural remedy for acne. Cucumbers can provide hydration to dry skin and calm irritation and inflammation caused by acne. To get the full benefits of cucumbers, cut the cucumber into slices and apply them to the skin, allowing them to sit for 20-25 minutes. Use this in addition to other treatments for maximum results.

200.   If you are a woman, breakouts can get even worse around your time of the month. The extra stress gives acne an ample opportunity to appear more and the hormones that are changing at that

time allow skin to go off course. Try to stay as stress free as possible during your period.

201.   When your breakouts become red and inflamed due to irritation, use ice to bring the redness and swelling down, in much the same way that you would on an injury. Icing your acne for 10 minutes at a time, every hour or so should provide noticeable improvement in the color and inflammation.

202.   One of the worst things that you can do in your battle versus acne is popping your pimples. This not only will leave a scar that could last for a long time, but will spread your acne internally and cause future breakouts that will usually be more severe. Medicate your face and wait it out, as patience plays a big role in controlling acne.

203.   Often foods will be the culprit of the acne that you have on your skin. If you notice that a specific food is causing your acne, try to limit it as much as possible. Ice cream, milk, cheese and other dairy products have been shown to increase acne.

204.   Everything in life that you do should be in moderation, as this also applies to the foods that you put into your body. If you ever eat too

much, you will not only get an upset stomach, but the excess nutrients in your body can cause a flare up of acne. Always eat proportionally to maintain healthy skin.

205.   Make sure that you skin is always clean, and wash it well after sweating. Bring along a pack of moist towelettes if you know you will be out of reach of running water and skin cleansers. The wipes clean and sanitize quickly and easily. Avoid using wipes in place of your cleanser.

206.   In your battle against acne you should never purchase cheap products in a supermarket or drug store. Generally, these products do not have the best ingredients for your skin, as they contain fillers or chemicals. Spend a few bucks for top of the line acne products for a strong foundation to your skin care regimen.

207.   There are numerous products available that will promise to deal with the common affliction of redness in the facial skin. However, before purchasing check the ingredient label of the item you are considering buying. The best rule of thumb is the less ingredients in the product, the better it is. Any product containing aloe vera juice is already a winning formula to help tame this issue.

208.   To help improve your acne problem avoid excessive sun exposure. A small amount of sun exposure is healthy for the skin and a light tan will help to hide some of the redness associated with acne. Too much exposure to sunlight, however, will cause skin to shed more than normal, resulting in clogged pores and an eventual increase in acne.

209.   An important tip to consider concerning acne, is to try to keep your hair out of your face throughout the day. This is important because your hair may transfer dirt and oil to your face. This is especially true, when any sort of physical activity is involved.

210.   You can use the whites of eggs to make a mask or to treat individual pimples. Just keep a small covered dish of the egg whites in your refrigerator and when you notice a pimple, just dab it on. Keep it for no longer than three days or you will be putting rotten eggs on your face to treat your pimples.

211.   An important tip to consider concerning acne, is to introduce chromium into your current diet. This is beneficial because it will assist with any skin infections or future pimples that you

may have. This is something that you can take once a day with food. A possible positive side effect is that chromium assists with weight loss, as well.

212.   Make sure you remember to wash your face even when you are not in the middle of an acne breakout. It is important to get in a routine of washing your face regularly. Ideally, you will want to wash your face once every morning then again before you go to bed.

213.   A good wash if you suffer from serious acne is a mild solution of salt water. Salt water will clean the oils and dirt off of your skin in the same way a cleanser would, but without the detrimental drying effects of many commercials cleansers that are intended for acne treatment.

214.   Eating a healthy diet can help to keep your skin clear and fresh. Doing this will help you because dairy and meat products can contain harmful hormones that produce negative effects on your skin.

215.   One of the most important ways to avoid getting acne is to keep your hands away from your face. The oils and bacteria on your fingers can actually damage your skin and cause pores to

be clogged. Don't ever push on or irritate your face at all with your fingers.

216.   If you are using an acne product that is high in salicylic acid content, it is important to remember the strong effect that this can have on your skin. Always remember to use only the directed amount, as excessive use can inflame your skin and cause even more breakouts. If you are noticing excess peeling or irritation, reduce your use to every other day, instead of daily or semi-daily.

217.   If you have aspirin laying around you can try an aspirin mask for your acne. Crush up several pills and add just enough water to make a mask. Apply this to the skin for about ten minutes. The ingredients in the aspirin will reduce the swelling and redness.

218.   Clean your cell phone and house phones regularly to avoid acne breakouts. Gently clean the screen and number pad with a damp cotton swap and some rubbing alcohol. This will remove any left over bacteria and oils from the surface and won't reapply them to your cheek and ear, when you go to talk.

219.   If you have acne, one of the best things that you can do is to refrain from thinking about your condition during the course of the day and night. Constant stress leads to an overproduction of oil, which can hurt your chances of tackling your issue and achieving a clear face.

220.   If acne has become a problem then you may want to realistically start looking at products like proactive. Proactive works by controlling the PH level of your skin and as such creates an environment inhospitable to bacterial growth. It is important with proactive however to be consistent with it's use as non-routine use results in minimal results.

221.   Small breakouts can be easily treated with spot treatment rather than an overall application of medicine. This can help prevent dry skin on the rest of your face. Some ingredients to look for in treatments are sulfur, salicylic acid or benzoyl peroxide. Hit the internet to find even more natural remedies.

222.   If you wear glasses or sunglasses you should wash them frequency if your skin is susceptible to acne. The frames on glasses can spread oil around the face and collect bacteria. The oil can then block pores on the skin and bacteria can

enter the pores and causes pimples, whiteheads, blackheads and cysts.

223.   In order to prevent breakouts, try to incorporate more Zinc into your diet. It is necessary for the skin's oil producing glands and an essential antibacterial mineral. It is proven that a person whose diet is low in Zinc is more likely to develop both acne and blackhead outbreaks on their face.

224.   Try using Tea Tree oil on a cotton ball or cotton swab to apply it to your pimples. The oil will kill the bacteria that cause the pimples and will clear-up the blemishes quite quickly. It is a great natural treatment for any kind of acne blemishes that you may have.

225.   Reducing the amount of dairy products and red meat in your diet, can help fight acne. Both of these foods require a lot of energy to digest. When the digestive system is working full-blast, excess waste products wind up backing up throughout the body, including in the skin. These wastes are significant contributors to acne problems.

226.   An important tip to consider when concerning acne is to consider using

Hydrocortisone as a remedy. This is an over the counter medication that has been proven to eliminate redness in acne. Be sure to not overuse this product, or use on unaffected areas so that you do not irritate your skin.

227. Crush uncoated aspirin tablets and mix with water and then apply this mixture to the face to create an aspirin mask. Keep the aspirin mask on for about ten minutes. Aspirin contains salicylic acid that helps fade acne scars and helps to prevent future breakouts. When using an aspirin mask, aspirin can be absorbed into your bloodstream, so consult with your doctor before starting this skin care regiment.

228. Many younger adults struggle with seborrhea, a skin condition which causes a thickened or increased production of sebum, or facial oils. Unlike acne, seborrhea is accompanied with thick, scaly patches. Look for topical treatments that contain zinc or coal-tar. These ingredients cut oil production without causing the skin to become thinner over time.

229. Buying an oil-free, dermatologist-approved moisturizer is essential for reducing acne. With the right oil-free moisturizer you can experience smooth skin without the side effect of additional

acne. If you do not use an oil-free moisturizer, there is a much greater chance your pores will get clogged and, thus, lead to a breakout of acne.

230.   It is a bad idea to pop pimples. It may seem relieving, but resist the temptation. Popping zits spreads more oil onto the skin, increasing the chances of additional outcroppings of acne arising later. Instead, use a wash or cream containing benzoyl peroxide and the acne will go away soon thereafter.

231.   If you are using an acne product that is high in salicylic acid content, it is important to remember the strong effect that this can have on your skin. Always remember to use only the directed amount, as excessive use can inflame your skin and cause even more breakouts. If you are noticing excess peeling or irritation, reduce your use to every other day, instead of daily or semi-daily.

232.   To get rid of a noticeable zit faster, you can apply baking soda or toothpaste containing baking soda on it. Leave this paste overnight on your skin: it might burn at first but it will help your zit develop faster. Make sure you thoroughly clean your skin the next day.

233. You can prevent acne by using sunscreen on a daily basis. Make sure that you don't stay in the sun for too long. Sunscreen will help your skin in the long run by avoiding damage that can be caused by the sun. Apply sunscreen to your skin in all seasons.

234. When it comes to acne, you are the best person in the world to know how your skin behaves. If your skin feels like it is getting oily, you should wash it immediately. If you feel it is becoming too dry, grab a moisturizer and massage gently on your face.

235. Resist the temptation to pop your acne pimples. While it may seem like an easy way to get rid of the pimple, you can spread the bacteria to other areas of your face, causing even more breakouts. Also, by breaking the skin's surface in this way, you may develop scarring.

236. Sometimes acne can be severe and you need to seek treatment from a licensed Dermatologist. Your Dermatologist can prescribe medications, skin care products, and surgery which would not be available over the counter. Seeking treatment sooner, rather than later, can allow for the most effective cure.

237.   Add a dab of toothpaste onto a stubborn zit before you go to bed at night. The toothpaste will dry out during the night, drying the zit along with it. Make sure that you first clean and pat dry the area before applying and always use toothpaste and not a gel.

238.   Try holding your cell phone or house phone away from your cheek when talking. This will help you avoid reapplying the dirt and bacteria from your phone back onto your skin, which can clog pores and cause acne. This may seem hard, but after a few practices, it will be second nature.

239.   Acne is a natural bodily response. You should never invest in a product that you see on the internet or that you see on TV that guarantees your acne will go away in an hour. These products almost always are all hype, which will leave you without money and with acne.

240.   Those who have a tendency to suffer from acne outbreaks should use care when selecting the temperature of water which is used for washing their skin. It is important to avoid washing the skin with hot water. Taking hot baths or long, hot showers can remove moisture from the skin, which can lead to the affected area becoming even more inflamed.

241.   An important tip to consider when concerning acne is that over washing can actually lead to more acne. This is important to consider because acne can cause you to feel unclean and the usual response is to wash yourself more frequently. This can be counterproductive as your skin may produce more oil to account for dryness.

242.   An important tip to consider when concerning acne is to try using a mixture of milk along with nutmeg directly on the area of concern. This is a great natural way to remove acne from your skin. Apply enough of each ingredient in order to make a paste-like texture.

243.   Use baking soda and water to help dry your acne up. Just mix the two ingredients and apply directly to any blemishes. Allow the mixture to dry for at least fifteen minutes and wash. Baking soda will help to neutralize the pH levels in your skin and can clear a blemish up fast.

244.   It is a good idea to wash your face with each night before you go to bed. Throughout the day, small particles of dust and dirt can accumulate on your skin, and if left on during the night, can

contribute to facial acne. Choose a cleanser that is best suited for your skin type.

245.   IF you suffer from severe acne and no treatment has ever worked, you may want to see a dermatologist and ask for an accutane prescription. Accutane is the strongest acne drug available and can successfully clear your skin when nothing else has worked. Accutane has a number of very serious side effects, so it should only be used as a last resort.

246.   If you wear make-up or a cleanser that is oil based, stop using it! These oil based products are horrible for acne. Since your body already produces oils naturally, adding more oils to your skin will only serve to increase your chances of developing acne problems. Instead, look for oil free products.

247.   Keep yourself hydrated to help with acne breakouts. Try to drink at least eight glasses of water a day to maintain clear skin. Water flushes out the toxins in your body, which also includes your skin. Not only will your skin be free from acne-causing toxins, but it will be able to retain the correct amount of moisture, to give it a healthier glow.

248.   Try not to touch your face as much. Your hands contain oils and your fingers, especially. Extra oil can clog pores on your face and cause pimples. Touching your face might not cause acne, but it can definitely exacerbate it. Try to break any habits that involve resting your head against your hand.

249.   A clear cut way to keep your face clear of acne, is to make sure that you wash your face daily, to keep your skin clean and refreshed. Make sure to wash with warm water and soap. Using hot water will burn the skin and cause damage.

250.   One way to prevent the clogging of pores is to use a blackhead remover. It is a little metal stick that you can purchase at any drugstore that you slide over your skin to remove any dirt or bacteria that is lodged in your pores. It is very easy to use and better than using your fingers.

251.   If you are a girl with acne, you should get birth control pills. Birth control pills regulate the hormones in your body and for most people, they reduce your acne considerably in just a few months. Ask your doctor about what kind of birth control pills has the best result on acne.

252.	Make sure that you are drinking plenty of water if you are suffering from acne. You skin needs to stay hydrated. If your skin becomes dehydrated, it is harder for your dead skin cells to shed. This can cause your pores to become blocked, and you could end up with more acne.

253.	Tretinoin, a topical retinoid, is a popular medication used to treat comedonal acne, blackheads and whiteheads. It is the acid form of vitamin A and works by increasing skin cell turnover and clearing blocked pores. The medication is available in cream or gel from under the following brand names: Stieva-A, Aberela, Atralin, Airol, Retin-A, Avita, Refissa and Renova.

254.	Shaving serves as exfoliation and therefore, can be an excellent way of removing dead skin cells. This can help to both prevent acne, and keep it from spreading if a break out has occurred. Avoid shaving any areas that are sore or infected however, as this can further irritate the skin.

255.	Working out is beneficial for the body, but it can often cause more breakouts. If you are prone to getting acne on your chest and back, switch to a body wash that contains salicylic acid. This is the main ingredient in several face washes. It will help unclog your pores.

256.   If you are looking for ways to prevent acne on your forehead or even the jaw line, it might help to keep your hair and hair products off these areas. The gels, mousses, hair sprays and other styling products could clog the pores on your face, which could lead to your face breaking out.

257.   Keep your hair out of your face the best you can. You hair carries a lot of oil and bacteria that can transfer to your face with contact. This can be a great reason for a breakout to develop. An easy solution is keeping your hair short or pulling it back with a ponytail holder.

258.   If you wear glasses or sunglasses you should wash them frequency if your skin is susceptible to acne. The frames on glasses can spread oil around the face and collect bacteria. The oil can then block pores on the skin and bacteria can enter the pores and causes pimples, whiteheads, blackheads and cysts.

259.   Salicylic acid, when used regularly can better prepare your skin to battle the blockages that lead to pimples. It is a fairly inexpensive agent

which removes the outer most layer of skin, along with all the pore clogging sediment that accumulates on it. Add salicylic acid to your daily routine to improve the overall process of cellular regeneration.

260.   The scars acne leaves behind can be removed through the process of dermabrasion. This is a serious procedure that should only be undertaken with the guidance of a dermatologist. Also, dermabrasion can severely irritate the skin, which makes it vulnerable to acne. Dermabrasion should only be used once acne problems have been resolved.

261.   Stop using products that have chemicals or perfumes in them on your hair, too! Even if you have stopped using these types of products on your skin, you can still get acne from the stuff you're using on your hair. Make sure to only use natural products on everything that touches your skin, even laundry detergent or fabric softener can cause your skin to become infected.

262.   An important tip to consider when concerning acne on your back is to be sure that you wear loose fitting clothing. This is important because it will allow for your skin to breathe and for air to get between your clothing and your

skin. Otherwise, the sweat, oil and dirt from your skin may clog up your pores.

263.   To prevent redness caused by acne, you shouldn't use a facial mask more than once a week. While masks are very good for your skin, you don't want to overdo it. They can actually cause more harm than good if used too much. They will dry out your skin and your body will produce more oils, causing breakouts.

264.   Regular exercise can be helpful when you're dealing with re-occurring acne problems. Exercise is a great way to release toxins, cleanse the pores (through sweating), and it also helps to relieve stress (which some believe contributes to acne). Stick to natural cotton exercise gear however, as synthetics can trap sweat and bacteria.

265.   Wash your face every night without fail, so you can avoid breakouts. This is especially true for women who wear makeup at night. If you do not wash your face before you go to bed, the oil, dirt and makeup sitting on your skin will be absorbed in your pores and can directly cause acne.

266.   Prevent breakouts with this easy tip. Clean your cellphone (and desktop phone at work) thoroughly with an alcohol wipe each day to take off excess oils. When you press your face against these objects, your pores can become clogged with old residue. When you don't clean these devices, you put yourself at risk to breakouts.

267.   If you're looking to get ride of acne as an adult, try a medication different from the ones targeted towards teenagers. A lot of acne medication developed for teenagers is formulated for lessening the appearance of large pimples overnight, and can be harsh to sensitive skin. Look for formulations made for adults, which usually contain sulfur as the active acne fighting ingredient.

268.   If you have very severe acne that is thick and painful, visit a dermatologist and ask about medication options. There are topical and oral medication options. Some medications can eliminate the oil producing glands underneath your skin. Discuss the options with your doctor and weigh the pros and cons of each choice.

269.   The sun is your enemy when you are fighting an acne problem. Stay in the shade, wear a hat and if you must get into the sunshine, wear a

powerful sunscreen. Be on guard against reflected light that bounces off water and other shiny surfaces on the brightest days, too. Staying out of the light will help your acne heal.

270.   An important tip to consider when concerning acne is knowing where acne can occur on your body. This is important in order to distinguish acne from other ailments. Acne will commonly occur on your face, and other times it may show up on the neck, chest, back, or your shoulders. It technically can occur in other places that may have clogged pores, but this would be more likely to occur from bad hygiene.

271.   If you wash your face at night and you notice a big pimple that is staring at you, try to ice it down before you go to bed. Just hold an ice cube on it for a few minutes and you may find that it does not look as swollen and red by the time you get out of bed in the morning.

272.   A honey mask can do wonders to cure an acne prone face. Honey has antibacterial properties and can be a soothing solution to even the worst acne break outs. It is also a very gentle product to use on sensitive skin. Use the mask once or twice a week for best results.

273.   If you experience discoloration in your skin after your acne goes away, use moisturizer on that area. Your skin can dry out and become scaly and lighter after your acne goes away. This is especially noticeable with people who have darker skin. Apply moisturizer to the area regularly to help the color return to normal.

274.   To decrease acne, be sure to intake at least two liters of water daily. When you do not drink enough water, your body does not shed its dead skin cells at the level that it should. These skin cells can block your pores and increase the level of acne you have.

275.   Get up off the couch and exercise! Exercise is a big trigger to decreasing acne. Not only is it a great stress reducer, but also, the increased blood flow also helps in the acne healing process. Plus, exercise helps your entire body to be healthy, which aids it in ridding itself of waste more efficiently and, in the long run, decreasing acne.

276.   A great tip for reducing or preventing acne is to make sure that your diet contains healthy amounts of fruits, vegetables, nuts, and seeds. There are a vast number of vegetables and other foods that have properties that fight acne.

Consider mixing these types of food by blending them into a tasty smoothie.

277.   To help you control your acne, a key piece of advice is to avoid touching the area on your body that is affected, especially with dirty hands. The bacteria and grease from your hands will further irritate the acne, which will not help decrease its size. If proper skin care is practiced and the acne is not touched, it should eventually disappear.

278.   Remind yourself not to pop your pimples with your fingers, or rest your cheek, chin or any other part of your face in your hand. Touching your hands to your face spreads bacteria to other parts of your face, and can cause more breakouts or infection. Infection can cause scarring or deep pitting that may only be helped by a skin specialist.

279.   If you have acne prone skin, change your pillowcase frequently. Over time, dirt and oil from your hair and skin can build up on your pillowcase. When you lay your face down on it at night it can then clog your pores, leading to acne. The best way to avoid this problem is by regularly changing your pillowcase.

280.　One wonderful, delicious way to get rid of acne is to substitute more fruit into your diet. This proven method will help your face clear up in no time. You can make smoothies for breakfast or lunch or just mix in some strawberries into your salad to make a fantastic dinner.

281.　If you are a woman, breakouts can get even worse around your time of the month. The extra stress gives acne an ample opportunity to appear more and the hormones that are changing at that time allow skin to go off course. Try to stay as stress free as possible during your period.

282.　Putting lemon juice onto a cotton ball or cotton swab and applying the juice directly onto an acne scar or pimple, can be a great natural acne remedy. The citric acid dries out pimples and lightens red marks and scars. For sensitive skin, try diluting the lemon juice with water or honey before applying.

283.　If you are experiencing a hard time ridding yourself of acne, try some skin care products that are made with natural products. Many commercially prepared skin care products contain harsh, irritating ingredients that can exacerbate skin problems. When your skin produces more oil, the pores get blocked which is what causes acne. Some natural products have an antibacterial effect, which can heal the skin.

284.   If back acne is an issue for you, then you may want to change your body cleanser. Opt for cleansers that contain salicylic acid or those geared toward clearing up acne and use these when you shower, once a day. Also, be sure to shower soon after vigorous exercise or physical activities, to avoid having the dirt and bacteria clog up your pores.

285.   Avoid stress to keep your face clear of unsightly bumps. Stress wakes up the hormones in the body that create acne. Keep yourself calm to keep your skin calm. Try deep cleansing breathes or taking time out for something you enjoy. The less stress you put your body through the more your skin will thank you.

286.   Mix lemon juice, yogurt, milk and honey together in a dish. Apply it to your face and let it sit for about twenty minutes. Rinse your skin thoroughly. Do this daily and you will see a reduction in the amount of acne that you have. It is one of the best natural face masks to treat acne.

287.   An important tip to consider when concerning acne is to consider taking a multi-vitamin supplement in addition to a healthy diet. This is important because acne can be a sign of many things, with malnutrition being one of them. If your body has all the nutrients it needs, then your skins natural oils will balance out.

288.   If your doctor has prescribed an antibiotic or medicine for the control of your acne, make sure you take the medicine in its entire course before deciding if it is working or not. Often, acne will get worse at the beginning of a new regimen as pimples come to the surface that were not visible before. Give your body ample time to adjust to the medicine before deciding on whether to continue treatment.

289.   An important tip to consider when concerning acne is to avoid drastic temperature changes with foods and beverages. This is important because too hot or cold temperatures can actually cause acne to occur around the mouth. This is not something that common, however it is something to watch out for if nothing else works.

290.   Crush uncoated aspirin tablets and mix with water and then apply this mixture to the face to

create an aspirin mask. Keep the aspirin mask on for about ten minutes. Aspirin contains salicylic acid that helps fade acne scars and helps to prevent future breakouts. When using an aspirin mask, aspirin can be absorbed into your bloodstream, so consult with your doctor before starting this skin care regiment.

291.   Make sure you get an adequate amount of sleep every night to help prevent breakouts. Strive to receive at least 6 hours, preferable 8, of sleep in order to give your body a change to cleanse your system of toxins. Without enough rest your body will not be able to flush out harmful waist from your skin which can result in a breakout.

292.   During breakouts, stay away from tight fitting apparel. Tight clothes can place pressure on blemishes and surrounding areas, thus causing more acne in the areas surrounding the initial blemish. So instead, during breakouts, wear loose fitting clothing that allows your skin to breathe. You will find that your breakouts will heal much quicker.

293.   Lowering the amount of dairy products in your diet can help reduce acne issues. Dairy products contain hormones that consequently

increase your own hormone levels. Increased hormone levels have a direct correlation with increased acne levels. Many people also have some level of lactose intolerance. When these people consume dairy products, the intolerance may manifest itself as acne. Therefore, if your daily diet consists of several dairy products, you should definitely consider removing some of them.

294.   To avoid the chances of creating more acne problems for yourself, avoid touching your face. Touching your face transfers dirt and bacteria to your pores, and can also cause already irritated areas to become even more irritated. Also avoid popping any pimples or blemishes with your bare fingers, as they will only make matters worse.

295.   A useful tip when dealing with acne is to be careful about the hair products you choose. Styling gels, sprays and other formulations containing oil, chemicals and scents have a tendency to drip and leech onto facial skin, which can lead to clogged pores. Using only the gentlest cleansers for the hair can also help keep excess oil at bay and away from the face.

296.   Another way you can improve your acne is to understand that it actually comes from what

you put into your body. Doctors have suggested that a low carb diet will reduce problem breakouts. Try to reduce the amount of breads and sugars that you are eating on a daily basis, and your face will thank you.

297.   Find a system to wash your face that works well for you. Not all are created equal, and some will irritate your skin more than they will soothe and clear it. Using the same system every day and keeping your skin clean and hydrated, will help your bodies natural defenses to attack and fight-off acne.

298.   Cutting back on your coffee intake can help to prevent acne. Coffee is linked to increased hormone levels in some individuals, which can trigger acne outbreaks. Eliminating or even reducing, the number of cups you drink a day, might have a positive effect on your complexion and overall, skin health.

299.   Consider using a cleaner rather than bar soap to clean your face. The skin's natural pH is 5.5, while bar soap typically has a pH of around 9. Bar soap can therefore alter the skin's pH enabling the types of bacteria that cause acne to multiply. Bar soap also contains thickeners which can block pores. Finally, bar soaps strip the skin

of all natural oils causing the sebaceous glands to overproduce oil leading to clogged pores.

300.   If you take antibiotics for acne, you may need to rebuild your body's defenses by using probiotics. Antibiotics don't just kill off bad bacteria; they also kill your body's friendly bacteria, which can cause more health problems down the road. Take a high-quality probiotic to rejuvenate your body's natural population of bacteria.

301.   If you have a case of acne, you need to wash the affected skin surface twice each day with acne soap. This soap has a sulfur base, and it is specially formulated to kill the bacteria that causes the acne and to aid in healing of the skin. Make sure when you wash your skin with this soap that you rub the affected area gently with a soft, clean cloth.

302.   If you want to prevent an acne breakout, you should clean sweat from your body immediately. Sweat will clog your pores, causing acne. After a heavy, sweat-inducing activity, take a good, hot shower.

303.   If you are prone to facial acne trouble, always cover your face when you apply hairspray

or other hair care products. Hair treatments that overrun onto the face help clog pores, giving your acne a boost you do not want it to have. This effect is common with even the most gentle, natural hair care products, so remember to cover up.

304.   A clean and natural look is best if your skin is prone to acne. Makeup can clog pores and cause more pimples, even when you're just trying to hide the ones you already have. Makeup applicators, such as sponges and brushes, tend to spread the bacteria. Throw out any applicators you are currently using and don't apply makeup again until your skin is totally zit-free.

305.   Many younger adults struggle with seborrhea, a skin condition which causes a thickened or increased production of sebum, or facial oils. Unlike acne, seborrhea is accompanied with thick, scaly patches. Look for topical treatments that contain zinc or coal-tar. These ingredients cut oil production without causing the skin to become thinner over time.

306.   If you wear glasses or sunglasses, always make sure you clean them. Cleaning them will remove the dirt or oil that could potentially cause acne or irritations on your skin. The oil, dirt, and

bacteria clogs pores and is the major cause of acne. Putting clean glasses on your face can help stop acne.

307.   Get up off the couch and exercise! Exercise is a big trigger to decreasing acne. Not only is it a great stress reducer, but also, the increased blood flow also helps in the acne healing process. Plus, exercise helps your entire body to be healthy, which aids it in ridding itself of waste more efficiently and, in the long run, decreasing acne.

308.   If you want to get rid of your acne quickly, try combining aspirin with lemon juice. Crush the aspirin and mix it with a little lemon juice. Put the liquid on your blemishes and leave it on overnight. Aspirin has a certain type of acid in it that helps your skin heal. Lemon juice has similar healing qualities.

309.   If you have acne or pimples underneath on or near your armpits, you may want to avoid scented deodorants. These kinds of deodorants prevent acne healing under the armpits and can actually cause the acne to spread. Try to find a deodorant that is lightly scented or not scented at all.

310.   Exfoliation is key to avoiding acne. Skin cells die naturally, but when they are not cleaned off of your face properly through exfoliation, they can lead to a buildup of oil and clog your pores, which leads to a breakout of acne. Use a face wash or scrubbing tool, that will properly exfoliate your skin.

311.   Chamomile is very efficient against acne. A tea bag that has been cooled down can reduce redness if it is placed on the affected area.

312.   If you do not understand where your acne comes from, get checked for allergies. Acne is a natural occurrence, but for some people it might be caused by certain chemicals. For instance, a laundry soap or a cleaning product can cause your skin to break out. If this is the case, try other brands.

313.   If you have developed acne scars a great effective cure is using medicated and non-medicated lotions. These lotions are easily applied privately at home and prove to be most helpful when used over a long period of time. Medicated lotions will help soften your skin over time and heal/treat existing scar tissue.

314.   If you have aspirin laying around you can try an aspirin mask for your acne. Crush up several pills and add just enough water to make a mask. Apply this to the skin for about ten minutes. The ingredients in the aspirin will reduce the swelling and redness.

315.   If you're fighting acne, check your moisturizers for ingredients that can make acne worse or prolong breakouts. Many rich or heavy moisturizing creams have ingredients that can clog pores, like sodium lauryl sulfate, cetearyl alcohol, cocoa butter or wheat germ oil. Other moisturizers contain ingredients like salicylic acid or retinol that can irritate skin that's trying to heal. Make sure to choose moisturizers that are non-comedogenic (non-clogging), non-acnegenic, and gentle on acne-prone skin.

316.   If you drink water often, try to add a few drops of lemon to your drink. Lemon acts as a powerful antioxidant, to help heal the internal components of your body that are contributing to acne. Drinking lemon water every day can help fight acne at its core and increase the vibrancy in your skin.

317.   If you are using acne fighting topical products, make sure to use a good moisturizer as

well. The ingredients that help to fight acne can also be extremely drying on your skin. If you suffer from oily skin, try using a gel based moisturizer and if you have dry skin use one that is cream or lotion based.

318. Purifying the blood is a great way to prevent acne breakouts. You can do this naturally by drinking a cup of Burdock root tea. Drink this tea three times a day and it will increase your blood circulation and purify your blood. This should lead to clearer skin and keep it clear in the future.

319. Some kinds of make-up contain a lot of harsh chemicals that can irritate skin cells and cause your skin to break out with acne. Using little to no make-up is best, but for those who like to wear make-up, there are many different brands available that are all natural and are less likely to cause problems with your skin.

320. If you have acne, rather than scrubbing your face, cleanse your face gently instead. Your skin is actually a protective layer. If you scrub it too harshly, you will aggravate your acne condition. Acne is frequently caused by genetic conditions that you cannot control, so any amount of scrubbing will not improve it.

321.   If your doctor has prescribed an antibiotic or medicine for the control of your acne, make sure you take the medicine in its entire course before deciding if it is working or not. Often, acne will get worse at the beginning of a new regimen as pimples come to the surface that were not visible before. Give your body ample time to adjust to the medicine before deciding on whether to continue treatment.

322.   If you plan on going out in the sun and you use acne medication, do not leave the house without oil-free sunscreen! Certain prescriptions and over-the-counter treatments can make skin even more sensitive to the sun, leading to sunburns and peeling which can worsen acne. A light sunscreen will help prevent further damage to your skin.

323.   If you have acne and long hair, pull your hair back in a ponytail. This is especially important when you exercise. The excess sweat coming from your hair can cause your oil producing glands to overreact. Having hair in your face also allows extra bacteria to build up.

324.   For controlling acne, don't use face washes or cleansers with oil or perfumes in them. Oil in

these products can clog pores and cause new pimples to appear. Perfumes are not advised because they can burn or irritate the already sensitive, delicate skin associated with acne.

325.	If you are a woman suffering from acne, consider taking birth control pills. If your acne is caused by high levels of hormones, such as testosterone and androgen, a prescription for a birth control pill could really help to clear your skin. Birth control pills regulate hormone levels, but make sure you ask your physician about any potential side effects.

326.	Are you struggling with severe acne? Try taking Isotretinoin! Isotretinoin is packaged under a variety of brand names, and it is a proven treatment for serve acne. The drug can dramatically reduce the severity and number of future acne breakouts. Unfortunately, the drug does have some scary potential side effects - such as birth defects - in pregnant woman.